Part one

Sickle Cell Disorder and Guidelines on Self-Management of Sickle Cell Disorder.

Dioscovite Natural Alternative for Sickle Cell Anaemia.

Hydroxyurea treatment for Sickle Cell Disease.

What is Sickle cell disease?

Sickle cell disease is a group of disorders that affects haemoglobin, the molecule in red blood cells that delivers oxygen to cells throughout the body. People with this disorder have a typical haemoglobin molecules called haemoglobin S, which can distort red blood cells into sickle or crescent shape.

Causes of Sickle Cell Disease.

Sickle cell disease is passed from parents to a child. A child is given 2 abnormal genes for haemoglobin, 1 from each parent.

Sickle cell disease usually requires lifelong treatment. Children and adults with sickle cell disease are supported by a team of different healthcare professionals working together at a specialist sickle cell centre.

What are the types of Sickle Cell Disease?

There are many different forms of sickle cell disease:

- Sickle cell anaemia, which includes Sickle Cell disease type SS and type sickle beta zero (SBO) thalassemia.
- Sickle cell disease type SC
- Sickle cell disease type sickle beta plus (SB+) thalassemia
- Sickle cell disease type SD, SE, and other sickle cell disease variants

What are the signs and symptoms of sickle cell disease?

The signs and symptoms of sickle cell disease are caused by the sickling of red blood cells. When red blood cells sickle they break down prematurely, which can lead to anaemia. Anaemia can cause shortness of breath, fatigue, and delayed growth and development in children. Yellowing of the eyes and skin is caused by the rapid breakdown of the red blood cells which are signs of jaundice.

The following symptoms may come and go, may happen during a sickle cell crisis:

- Headaches
- Pale skin
- Low energy

- Shortness of breath
- Pain anywhere in your body

Painful episodes can occur when sickled red blood cells, which are stiff and inflexible, get stuck in small blood vessels. These episodes deprive tissues and organs of oxygen-rich blood and can lead to organ damage, especially in the lungs, kidneys, spleen, and brain. A particular serious complication of sickle cell disease is high blood pressure in the blood vessels that supply the lungs (pulmonary hypertension). Pulmonary hypertension occurs in about one-third of adults with sickle cell disease and can lead to heart failure.

What problems can sickle cell disease cause?

Sickle cell disease can cause:

- Anaemia – When you have fewer red blood cells to carry oxygen in your body, which can make you feel tired.
- Pain crisis – pain in your chest, stomach, or bones. This happens when sickle cells block your blood vessels.
- Acute chest syndrome – a lung problem that happens when sickle cells block the blood vessels in your lungs. This can be life threatening and you will need to go to the hospital.
- Organ damage –harm to important organs like your brain, heart, lungs, kidneys and eyes. This can lead to serious problems like kidney failure or vision loss.

Sickle cell disease can even shorten life – but hydroxyurea can help you live longer. That is why it is important to consider taking it.

What is a sickle cell crisis?

A sickle cell crisis is pain that can begin suddenly and last several hours to several days. It happens when sickled red blood cells block small blood vessels that carry blood to your bones. You might have pain in your back, knees, legs, arms, chest or stomach. The pain can be throbbing, sharp, dull or stabbing. How often and how bad the pain gets varies a lot from person to person and from crisis to crisis.

You might be able to treat your pain crisis at home with medicines that you take by mouth. If these medicines don't control your pain, you can't keep fluids down or you know that you are having severe pain, you might need to be treated in the emergency department. If your pain still isn't controlled or you have other problems, you might need to be treated in the hospital.

What causes a sickle cell crisis?

Most of the time, you won't know what caused your sickle cell crisis. A crisis usually has more than one cause. However, you can do severally things that might keep a crisis from occurring.

- Don't drink a lot of alcohol.
- Don't smoke. If you do smoke quit.
- Exercise regularly but not so much that you become really tired. When you exercise drink lots of fluids.
- Drink at least eight 12-ounce glasses of water a day during warm weather.
- Reduce or avoid stress. Talk to your doctor if you are depressed or have problems with your family or job.
- Treat any infection as soon as it occurs. When in doubt, see your doctor.

- Wear warm cloths outside in cold weather and inside in air-condition rooms during hot weather. Also, don't swim in cold water.
- Try to be positive about yourself.
- Tell your doctor if you think you might have a sleep problem, such as snoring or if you sometimes stop breathing during sleep.
- If you have another medical condition, like diabetes, get treatment and control the condition.
- If you are pregnant or plan to become pregnant get early pregnant care.
- Only travel in commercial airplanes. If you have to travel in an unpressurized aircraft, talk to your doctor about extra precautions.

What can I use at home to control my pain?

Some over the counter medicines might help relieve mild pain. Taking acetaminophen (brand name: Tylenol) or aspirin might help. Medicine like ibuprofen might help if you can safely take these medicine. However, talk to your doctor before you take any medicine for your pain.

If you have moderate to severe pain your doctor might prescribe a mild narcotic like codeine. This medicine is often given with aspirin or acetaminophen. You take this medicine regularly around the clock, rather than waiting for the pain to return before taking your next dose.

A heating pad, hot bath, rest or message might help. Physical therapy to relax and strengthen your muscles and joints might lessen your pain. Self-hypnosis and activities to keep you from thinking about your pain such as watching television, playing video games or talking on the telephone might also help.

It is important for you to have a positive attitude, create a supportive environment and develop coping skills to help you deal with your disease.

Work with your family doctor to set goals for the management of your pain. Becoming more actively involved in your treatment will help you better manage your health condition.

Guidelines on Self-Management of sickle cell Disorder.

Lifestyle Issues

- Face your future or your affected child's future with optimism. Do not despair.

- Dress appropriately for cold weather and for cold air-conditioned offices. Limit exposure to sudden changes in temperature, especially from warm to cold weather.

- Keep dry, especially during the rainy season. Always carry an umbrella, raincoat, and rain boots during the wet season.

- If beaten by the rain, change as soon as possible into dry clothes, have a warm drink (non-alcoholic) and move around the house. Do not go to bed straightaway.

- Avoid stress- physical, emotional and mental stress.

- Avoid long aeroplane journeys when you are unwell. If you develop sickle cell crisis on board an aeroplane report to the cabin crew and ask for oxygen and painkillers.

- Eat what you like provided it is balanced and contains carbohydrates, proteins, fats, vegetables and fresh fruits daily. The natural vitamins in fresh fruits and vegetables have been shown to be of superior nutritional value to those sold as pills or lotions. Eat one egg per day.

- Drink at least 3 litres of water (plain or sweetened with fruit juices etc.) every day. If you bed wet at night, please do not drink after say 7pm and ensure you urinate just before going to bed. A child should drink about 50 ml per kg body weight daily. Manufactured soft drinks with gas should be limited as excessive gas can cause distension, pain or discomfort in the abdomen.

- People with sickle cell disorder tend to accumulate iron in their bodies and excess of iron can be harmful to various organs. Never take blood tonics, iron or ferrous tablets or iron containing vitamin preparations unless your body iron status has been investigated and you have been diagnosed by a blood disease specialist (haematologist) to have iron deficiency anaemia in addition to sickle cell disorder.

- Be wary of, and avoid unproven herbal or synthesized 'wonder cures' widely advertised to separate you from your money. Ask your sickle cell doctor or Centre for advice.

- Good Personal and environmental hygiene is very important.

- Keep a diary of events, noting sites and duration of pain, medication used and their effects, prior events or other symptoms such as chills, rigors, fever (learn to measure your temperature), sore throat, etc. This record will help your doctors and other health care workers.

Limiting Anaemia

- Take one tablet of folic acid 2 mg- 5 mg once every day to prevent the folate deficiency which occurs in people with high turn-over of red blood cells (haemolytic anaemia) as in sickle cell disorder. By doing so, you prevent more severe anaemia.

  Folic acid (folate) is a vitamin that is needed to make new cells in the body, including red blood cells. The body does not store very much folic acid. You need a regular fresh supply to keep healthy. Many foods, containing folic acid, include spinach, sprouts, broccoli, green beans, peas, chickpeas, brown rice, kidney, liver and potatoes. A normal balanced diet contains enough folic acid. However, a lack of folic acid will cause anaemia and sometimes other symptoms. Multivitamins should be used but not with iron content.

Preventing infection

- Avoid exposure to mosquitoes as much as possible. Wear long sleeved shirts and trousers in the evenings and sleep under a chemically treated mosquito net at night to limit exposure to mosquito bites.

- To prevent malaria, take paludrine tablets 200mg daily. For children give paludrine tablet 50-100 mg daily according to age/weight.

- Influenza (Flu) is a seasonal virus infection. If you have sickle cell disorder, it is best prevented by receiving a Flu vaccination once a year.

- Pneumococcal bacteria commonly cause deadly infections in children with sickle cell disorder. Oral penicillin taken twice daily can prevent many of these infections. Give all children aged 2 months to 3 years, 125 mg penicillin twice daily.

Older children should take 250 mg twice daily. In addition, pneumococcal vaccinations should be given from the first year of life. Please seek expert opinion on the names, doses and frequencies of these life-saving vaccines. Other immunisations like for polio, tetanus, measles, whooping cough recommended to all children should also be taken.

Penicillin V

Because of poor splenic function and underdeveloped immunity, people with sickle cell disorder are more prone to infection and the pneumococcus is commonly implicated as the major cause of infection often leading to meningitis and pneumonia, which can be fatal especially in children under the age of five. Worldwide research has demonstrated that the daily use of a broad spectrum antibiotic, for example oral penicillin, significantly reduces mortality and morbidity.

Preventing Strokes

- Same as a heart attack is due to the interruption of blood supply to parts of the heart, a stroke (brain attack) is due to the interruption of blood supply to parts of the brain.
  A stroke may lead to partial or complete paralysis of limbs, fits and convulsions, speech difficulty, intellectual deficit or death.

- About 7 or 100 (7%) children with sickle cell disorder aged between 2 and 16 years will develop strokes and will go on to have further strokes if preventive measures are not applied. The initial stroke as well as further strokes can be prevented if the child receives a blood transfusion every 3 or weeks or takes a calculated dose of oral hydroxyurea daily.

The challenge is to identify the children who are likely to develop strokes so that they can be protected by applying one of these preventive measures.

- An ultrasound scan of the brain, using a transcranial doppler can identify children with a high risk of developing strokes. Therefore, all children aged 2 to 16 years should undergo a transcranial doppler scan to determine their stroke risk which if high, will qualify them for stroke prevention by blood transfusion or hydroxyurea. The prevention of an initial stroke is referred to as primary prevention. Secondary prevention is the prevention of further strokes in a child who already had a stroke.

Preventing or reducing the frequency of sickle cell Crisis

- Make a note of activities, climatic conditions or foods which tend to bring about your crisis or your child's crisis and learn to avoid them.

- Hydroxyurea (HU) is a chemotherapy medicine that has been used to treat many disorders, including sickle cell disease (SCD). Research has shown that patients with sickle cell disease who take hydroxyurea are admitted to hospital because of painful events only half has often as patients who do not take hydroxyurea, have fewer acute chest crisis and have less need for blood transfusion if they are admitted to hospital. Hydroxyurea, taken orally daily, can reduce the frequency of sickle cell pain crisis and prolong life. Discuss the role of hydroxyurea with a sickle cell specialist doctor. It can be risky unless taken under the supervision of a sickle cell specialist. In other words, it must never be self-medicated.

Control Sickle Cell Crisis

- As soon as the first pain is felt, take 2 tablets of paracetamol 500mg each and repeat the dose every 4 hours not exceeding 8 tablets per day. In addition, take ibuprofen tablets 600mg (in adults) every 8 hours until the pain subside. Do not take ibuprofen or a similar drug on an empty stomach. Eat some food first. If you weigh less than 50kg take only 400mg every 8 hours.

- Alternately, instead of the above, take 3 tablets of Parafen (it contains paracetamol + ibuprofen) thrice daily after meals or if you weigh less than 50kg take 2 tablets thrice daily.

- For children, as soon as the first pain is felt, give oral or rectal paracetamol and repeat the dose every 4 hours. Dose is 750mg for children aged 12-14 years; 500mg for ages 6-11 years: 250mg for ages 2-5 years and 125mg for children below 2 years. In addition, take ibuprofen tablets (or syrup) 400mg in adolescent and 200mg in children thrice daily with meals until the pain subsides.

- Alternately instead of the above give one tablet of Parafen (it contains paracetamol + ibuprofen) thrice daily after meals to children under 12 years and 2 tablets thrice daily to older children.

- To relieve early bone pain, hot fomentation followed by messaging the site or sites with gels or balms can be useful. Soak a towel in hot water and place it at the site of the pain for about 10 minutes (please avoid scalding yourself). Then message the site with a balm or gel containing salicylate, or ibuprofen or diclofenac. This can help to relieve early bone pain and prevent escalation.

- If you do not feel better within 24-36 hours or if you are very pale (i.e. anaemic) or breathless on slight exertion please consult a doctor immediately, preferably one experienced in the treatment of patients with sickle cell anaemia.

- If there is no relief or there is fever, consult your doctor as soon as possible. Do not assume that fever is always caused by malaria. It can be due to a viral or a bacterial infection.

- If your child is pale or breathing too fast or with difficulty seek medical attention immediately. Learn to recognise pallor, a sign of anaemia, and enlarged spleen as these signs demand urgent medical attention, preferably by someone experienced in the treatment of patients with sickle cell anaemia.

What Teachers, Nurses and Administrators can do to support students with Sickle Cell Disease?

1. Ensure adequate access to water/hydration

Staying well hydrated by drinking plenty of water can help prevent pain episodes and other health problems. Thus, unlimited access to water throughout the school day is essential. Frequent, small amounts of water are better than trying to drink a large amount of fluid at one time. Allowing access to a bottle of water in class is an option.

2. Allow frequent bathroom breaks

Children with sickle cell disorder produce large amounts of dilute urine even when they are dehydrated. Thus, they may need to go to the bathroom more often than other children. Do not restrict students with sickle cell disorder from bathroom breaks. Provide a special bathroom pass to limit disruptions in instruction and to minimize attention drawn to the student exiting the classroom.

3. Allow accommodations during extreme temperatures and conditions

Cold or hot weather can trigger pain crisis. Teachers should not assign a student with sickle cell disorder a seat in drafty locations, directly in front of fans or under air conditioner vents. Permit layered clothing in the classroom. Remind students with sickle cell disorder to wear a jacket outside during cold or rainy weather or to take off a layer of clothing when it is hot. They should not exercise in extreme conditions (e.g., avoid cold and high heat and humidity).

4. Allow accommodations during physical education and recess activities

Most children with sickle cell disorder can engage in moderate exercise, including running, jumping, and riding bikes. However, teachers may modify curricula so that a child experiencing health problems related to sickle cell disorder can participate in physical education in roles that are less strenuous, such as being the physical education teacher's "assistant," "storekeeper," or "umpire." Admitting fatigue, which may be due to anaemia, may be embarrassing or draw unwanted attention to a child with sickle cell disorder. Even with moderate activity, regular breaks or a brief period of rest after physical activity may be necessary. In addition, incorporate frequent water breaks into any physical activity plans. Teachers and administrators may want to consult with the child's parent or ask the child the level of activity they can tolerate during recess. Also, remember never require children with sickle cell disorder to exercise in cold weather without extra layers of clothing to keep warm.

5.Take special care of injuries

Never apply a cold pack to an injury or pain site if a child with sickle cell disorder is injured during the school day. However, other first aid measures are safe for children with sickle cell disorder who are injured at school. First aid measures that should be provided when necessary, include applying direct pressure for bleeding, wrapping with an ace bandage, or elevating a hurt limb.

6. Watch for signs of stroke

Some children living with sickle cell disorder may have learning difficulties due to health problems associated with stroke (blockage of blood vessels in the brain that then causes brain damage}. Strokes may be difficult to detect when they affect a small portion of the brain, but they are extremely important to watch for because they are relatively common in the early school years among children with sickle cell disease. Teachers should be aware that declines in academic achievement, inability to maintain attention, difficulties with organization and mild delays in vocabulary development may be due to small brain injuries caused by strokes. Moreover, teachers are in a unique position to notice changes in school performance that might indicate a stroke and should not simply assume that poor attention in the classroom is due to a lack of the child's motivation or desire to do well in school. Teachers should contact parents when changes in learning or a child's attentiveness are detected so that the child's doctor can be notified. Formal neurocognitive and educational testing may be necessary to determine any learning difficulties caused by stroke. The testing may help school personnel in developing the best teaching strategies for the student.

7. Be aware of emotional well-being

Not all children with sickle cell disorder have outward signs of illness. However, children with sickle cell disorder may be smaller in size, have delayed puberty or experience jaundice (yellowing of the skin and eyes). These sometimes subtle, outward signs may make children living with sickle cell disorder targets for teasing and bullying. Students with sickle cell disorder may cope with their differences by being aggressive, isolating themselves, or avoiding social situations with peers. Like other children with medical challenges, children with sickle cell disorder may not have as many opportunities to play with other children, thus recreational activities or group based classroom assignments may serve as opportunities for developing good interpersonal skills and boosting a student's self-esteem. Teachers can also help children identify special interests and talents that may help them identify career goals.

8. Maintain open communication with parents

Teachers can help create a positive relationship between home and school as well as a sense of community for students by maintaining open communication with a child's family through notes, e-mail, phone contact conferences to discuss the student's performance and well-being in the classroom and at home. Regular contact with a student's parents is especially important for children with a chronic illness. Some children with sickle cell disorder will have periods when they are unable to attend school, but may not be hospitalized. Whether a student is hospitalized or homebound due to health problems related to sickle cell disorder, teachers must allow students the opportunity to complete all the required work. Thus, it may be especially important for teachers to talk to parents about missed school plans prior to a period of illness (tutoring, assignment plan, a second set of books to keep at home or online resources for classwork). When devising makeup work for any child with a chronic medical condition, teachers may want to consider the quality of the assignment over the quantity. Finally, teachers and school nurses should keep up-to=date contact numbers for the student's parents and doctor in case of emergency.

Dioscovite Natural Alternative for Sickle Cell Anemia

Dioscovite is composed of nutrients that appear in food that has been eaten for centuries. One of these foods is the African Yam. The name Dioscovite is composed of two components: Dioscoria means Yam, and Vite which represents Vitamin. Therefore, Dioscovite is a coined name representing Yam Vitamin.

It is a wonderful product to try if you are looking to do something nutritional, and something that is not harmful to your body, and that is safe and nontoxic. It eliminates pain that you would have on a daily basis.

You should be taking Dioscovite every single day. It works best prophylactically meaning it's best taken to prevent sickling and stop sickle cell pain. The reason for this is that Dioscovite binds irreversibly to your Red Blood Cell Hemoglobin as it is being produced. Once it binds to the Hemoglobin, this prevents the cell from sickling. That cell is preserved. However, your bone marrow continued to produce more and more Red Blood Cells on a routine basis. The other Red Blood Cells being produced will still sickle unless Dioscovite binds to it. For this reason, Dioscovite should be taken on a daily continuous basis.

Dioscovite Mechanism of Action

As you probably know, those who suffer from Sickle Cell have a different type of Hemoglobin in their Red Blood Cells. This is called Hemoglobin S. Dioscovite works by undergoing a series of chemical reactions in the Red Blood Cell leading to a metabolite interacting with Hemoglobin S correcting the polarity that differentiates Hemoglobin S from normal Hemoglobin. By doing this, this prevents the Hemoglobin S from clumping together and leading to Sickled Cells. Once this occurs Hemoglobin S behaves like Hemoglobin A. Therefore, Dioscovite stops sickle cell crisis and sickle cell pain by attacking the problem at the molecular level.

One major issue to look out for is the bowel regimen. Dioscovite is absorbed mostly in the small and large intestine. Therefore, if excess stool is located in your intestines, the Dioscovite would be absorbed into the stool. The more absorbed into your stool, the less that is absorbed into your blood stream where your red blood cells are located. Without Dioscovite reaching your blood, your Hemoglobin sickles causing pain/complications.

That is why it is imperative to make sure you are regular. At a minimum you should be consuming at least 10 grams of fiber every day, and drinking at least 8 cups of water. This can be achieved utilizing fruits and vegetables. This is absolutely essential. If you don't get the full 10 grams of fiber through this route, it is recommended that you fill the gap with fiber supplements. Ensuring 4-6 mg of fiber consumed with your dinner works particularly well.

To ensure that your daily dose is absorbed maximally, it is recommended that you take it in the morning, after you have had your typical morning bowel movement. Its best to avoid any other medication within 2 hours. That way it will be maximally absorbed, and you can experience the best results.

Constipation is the number one issue affecting the efficacy of Dioscovite. Other potential issues may be anything that precipitates sickling. Dehydration, Alcohol (which causes Dehydration etc.), too much exposure to cold are others to watch out for.

Finally look for any new medication, new food, or new herbal remedy/supplement that you started newly. The body can react differently to any of the above. In order to stop sickle cell crisis. It is important to keep note of anything altering the health, and wholeness that should always be yours on Dioscovite.

What other vitamins and minerals should be taken with Dioscovite?

We recommend folic acid at least 2-5 mg per day. There are definitely other vitamins and minerals we recommend. An overview of them have been listed below. Remember that Dioscovite should be taken in water 2 hours before or after all vitamins and minerals.

- Folic Acid 2-5 mg per Day
- Diet with adequate Meat to ensure adequate Vitamin B12 intake
- Copper 2mg per Day

- Zinc 50mg-100 mg per Day (in the morning or early Afternoon. Zinc competes with Copper for absorption so Zinc should be taken at least 8 hours separately from Copper)
- Magnesium 250 mg per Day
- Selenium 100 mcg per Day
- Vitamin B6/B-complex
- Vitamin E

Hydroxyurea Treatment for Sickle Cell Disease.

Hydroxyurea is a medicine that can help children and adults with sickle cell disease. It is a medicine that doctors have used to treat people with sickle cell disease since the 1980s. The Food and Drug Administration (FDA) approved it for treating adults with sickle cell disease in 1998. In 2017, the FDA approved it to treat children with sickle cell disease. Research studies show that hydroxyurea lowers the following:

- The numbers of acute chest syndrome (pneumonia) events
- The number of pain crisis
- The need for blood transfusions
- The number of trips to the hospital

Hydroxyurea also might prevent damage to the spleen, kidneys, lungs, and brain.

Hydroxyurea is given by mouth one (1) time each day. It comes in liquid or capsule form.

Hydroxyurea is also used to treat cancer. But doctors use a lower dose (amount) to treat sickle cell disease than to treat cancer.

Which children should take hydroxyurea?

Hydroxyurea is considered for children who have had:

- Many painful events,
- Several cases of acute chest syndrome (pneumonia),
- Several anaemia or
- Other special problems with their internal organs.

How does hydroxyurea works?

Hydroxyurea makes your red blood cells bigger. It helps them stay rounder and more flexible and makes them less likely to turn sickle shape.

The medicine does this by increasing a special kind of hemoglobin called hemoglobin F. Hemoglobin F is also called fetal hemoglobin because new born babies have it. When you have higher levels of hemoglobin F, your red blood cells are less likely to cause problems.

Safety and Side Effects

Many people with sickle cell disease have taken hydroxyurea safely for over 20 years. Even young children can take it. There is no evidence that hydroxyurea causes cancer in people with sickle cell disease. It's been used safely since the 1980s.

All medicines can have side effects. Some people who take hydroxyurea may experience these side effects:

- Thinning hair or mild hair loss
- Fingernails beds that turn darker

- Nausea (feeling sick to your stomach)

Very rarely, hydroxyurea can cause more serious side effects. But most people with sickle cell disease who take hydroxyurea don't have any serious side effect.

If you have any new symptoms after you start taking hydroxyurea, tell your doctor – you may be able to take a lower dose.

Will I be able to start a family?

If you're thinking about having a baby, be sure to talk to your doctor about the pros and cons of taking hydroxyurea. Experts are still learning about how hydroxyurea affects your ability to have a healthy baby. Taking it during pregnancy is a personal choice that your doctor can help you make.

Women

- If you are pregnant or planning to get pregnant, talk to your doctor to make a plan.
- Hydroxyurea may increase the risk of birth defects, but we don't know for sure yet.
- Some women choose to stop taking hydroxyurea early in their pregnancy and then start it again during the third trimester (after 29 weeks).

Men

Hydroxyurea can lower your sperm count, which may already be low due to sickle cell disease.

Painful erections are a complication of sickle cell disease that can cause permanent damage to the penis. Hydroxyurea may make these painful erections less likely.

What do I need to know about taking Hydroxyurea?

Most people take hydroxyurea pills once a day. Your doctor will prescribe the dose he or she thinks is right for you. Sometimes you may need to take a different number of pills on certain days.

- Hydroxyurea is safe to take with most other medicines – but it is always a good idea to check with your doctor or pharmacist before starting a new medicine.
- Hydroxyurea pills are capsules that are about three-quarters (3/4) of an inch long.
- Hydroxyurea will only work if you take it every day.
- Missing a dose is not dangerous and will not reverse the benefit of the drug.

Checking your blood count

You'll need to get your blood cell counts checked regularly when you take hydroxyurea. When you first start taking it, you may need to get your blood counts checked every month.

Ask your doctor about your blood count numbers to see how they change. The changes in your blood count can be a good sign that the hydroxyurea is working!

These test will check for:

- Hemoglobin, the protein that carries oxygen in red blood cells. Hydroxyurea works by making your hemoglobin level go up.

- The size of your red blood cells (measured as 'mean cell volume" or MCV). Hydroxyurea works by making your red blood cells bigger.
- Neutrophils, a type of white blood cell. Hydroxyurea makes the number of neutrophils go down. This is okay as long as your white blood count doesn't get too low.

Your doctor might change your dose based on your blood cell counts. For example, if the neutrophils in your blood don't go down, your doctor might increase your dose.

Your doctor will also check to see if some types of blood cells get too low. If this is the case, your doctor might ask you to stop taking hydroxyurea for a while.

Hydroxyurea can help people with sickle cell diseases have fewer pain crisis and better health.

Part two

Our experience with sickle cell disorder, my daughter's Story.

Our Story

I got back from work and noticed my five months old daughter's hands were swollen. I did not understand what was happening, I asked my mother-in-law who was assisting me to look after my daughter during the day, what happened and why she allowed my baby to fall down. She said that my daughter did not fall down that she carried and monitored her throughout the day.

I took my daughter to the hospital the next day. The doctor immediately asked about my genotype and husband's genotype. I told the doctor that I am genotype AS and my husband's genotype was AA. He wanted to know if I was sure. I told him my husband showed me his laboratory result from school. My husband had always believed he was genotype AA from childhood. He told me that the swollen hands were sickle cell disorder sign called hand-foot syndrome and I should wait for my daughter to get to a year old before doing any laboratory test.

Hand-Foot Syndrome

Swelling in the hands and feet usually is the first symptom of Sickle Cell Disorder. This swelling, often along with a fever, is caused by the sickle cells getting stuck in the blood vessels and blocking the flow of blood in and out of the hands and feet.

People with sickle cell disease start to have signs of the disease during the first year of life, usually around 5 months of age. Symptoms and complications of sickle cell disease are different for each person and can range from mild to severe.

The reason that infants don't show symptoms at birth is because baby or fatal haemoglobin protects the red blood cells from sickling. When the infant is around 4 to 5 months of age, the baby or fetal haemoglobin is replaced by sickle haemoglobin and the cells begin to sickle.

The most common treatments for swelling in the hands and the feet are pain medicine and an increase in fluids such as water.

I was in denial

I was in shock and denial. I did not want to accept that my child had sickle cell disease. No, it is not possible. I serve a great God that cannot allow this to happen to my child. I wanted a second opinion so I took my daughter to a different hospital. The doctor told me the same thing the previous doctor told me.

We waited for her to clock a year old before conducting the laboratory test on my daughter Emma and the result came out genotype AA. I went to a different hospital after some weeks and conducted another test and the genotype test result came out as AA too. My husband and I were so happy and grateful to God. We thought the sickness was just minor infection which would varnish over time. Before now we used to be on hospital admission for days, she was always being treated for infection.

In the early years of her life, she really went through a lot. There was a day I came back very late from work and was about laying her on the bed when she started shivering and was almost convulsing, then I rushed her to the hospital in the mid-night. I had to call my boss and explained the situation of things to her. She had high temperature and was in pains. The doctors were trying to get veins to extract blood and also to pass water through. It took them time before they got a vein. She cried and I was crying too. The doctors and nurses kept telling me to be strong for her, but I could not stand her being in pains. We were in the hospital for days because her temperature was high. We were later discharged after some days.

At age two years

When Emma became two years, she fell ill again. We took her to the hospital and this time around the doctor conducted another genotype test and the result game out genotype SS. My husband and I were in shock and unhappy when we were informed. I blamed myself for putting my daughter through the ordeal. I went to work the next day miserable and unhappy. I was calling my mother-in-law at intervals to enquire about Emma. I was no longer joyful at work.

I worked in one of the commercial banks as a front desk officer for ten years. I could not cope at work anymore. The physical and emotional stress was too much for me. I fell ill at a time and couldn't walk. Series of test was conducted on me and they could not detect anything wrong with me. I was not okay in my body which I knew but the doctors kept telling me there was nothing wrong with me. They told me to avoid stress and apply for my annual leave. My mother was the one who assisted in taking me to see a specialist doctor, who prescribed some drugs for me that helped temporarily. I had to resign from work after two years for my sanity sake and also to concentrate on my daughter Emma who was in the hospital then on admission.

My daughter was in and out of different hospitals for treatment. There was a day in one of the hospitals I was thinking in my heart God why do you hate me so much, why did you allow this to happen to us. I would cry myself to sleep and have nightmares. I could not count the number of times she was in and out of hospital admission. There was another day I had to rush her to the hospital in the middle of the night, because she complained of pains in her stomach and arm.

They checked her blood level and noticed it was lower than her normal blood level, then they had to transfuse her. The student doctor who was to look for veins couldn't find veins in her hands. He kept poking her two feet with needle and my girl was crying in pains. I had to caution the doctor who got angry and left me with my daughter. The nurses in that hospital were so unprofessional gossiping in my native language saying in this day and age of advancement I allowed myself to be blinded by love by marrying a genotype AS man and given birth to sickle cell child. I ignored them because they don't know my story.

While my daughter was crying in pains, I was also shedding tears blaming myself. She was uncomfortable with the oxygen that was passed through her nose. At a point, my daughter was the one consoling me saying Mummy please don't cry, I will be okay. She is a strong girl and a warrior. I had to apologise to the student doctor who got another Doctor to locate the veins on her feet. We never went back to that hospital after the unprofessional manner we were treated.

Information is Power

A formal colleague who also had sickle cell disorder described the pain has someone using a table knife to cut or chop one severally in the arm. Emma has always wanted to swim in school because her elder sister swims in school on Fridays. My husband did not want her to feel left out so he instructed that the school should allow her to swim. She landed in the hospital after school that day because she was in pains. We never knew she was not supposed to swim at all.

After her first blood transfusion, we visited the sickle cell centre. Information is power. In the centre we were counselled and told what to do and what not to do. We ensure she takes enough water, eat balanced diet, bath with warm water, avoid swimming, take her routine drugs and sleeps under mosquito treated net at night.

The last time she was in the hospital, her temperature was high and fluctuating. We were in the hospital for ten days. They kept doing series of test and changing her medication. At a point I felt the doctors were confused and were experimenting with Emma. The doctors did not want to discharge us because her temperature was fluctuating. I had to sign at my own risk, before I was allowed to take her home. When we got home I gave her the drugs given to us from the hospital but the temperature was still fluctuating. I was just tired of crying and frustrated with the situation. Then I called my eldest daughter, my mother and I pick a bottle of anointing oil and anointed Emma and we each took turns to pray for her. It was like a miracle, she became instantly okay and was playing around the house and she has been okay ever since and has not stepped into the hospital since then.

There is Life and death in the power of the tongue

For verily I say unto you, that whatsoever shall say unto this mountain, be thou removed, and be thou cast into the sea; and shall not doubt in his heart, but shall believe that those things which he saith shall come to pass; he shall have whatsoever he saith.

Therefore, I say unto you, "what things so ever ye desire, when ye pray, believe that ye receive them, and ye shall have them. Mark 11: 23-24 King James Version Bible.

There is life and death in the power of the tongue. I started saying positive words to my child. I stopped being fearful. I started reading, listening and watching faith filled messages on my television and phone. I kept saying, Emma you shall not die but live to declare the glory of the Lord. You shall not die young, you have a great life, you are a testimony, you shall live to see your great grandchildren in good health and prosperity. You shall be the head and not the tail in Jesus name. Amen.

Say what you desire in your child daily. Your words are powerful. Have faith in God.

Anytime Emma wants to say anything negative, I rebuke her and tell to always say positive things. God created heaven and earth with words. There is power in our words. We have to always confess and declare what we desire daily.

My eldest daughter noticed we were giving Emma so much attention and felt insecure. We had to explain Emma's health condition to her and how she could also help in taking care of her younger sister. She adjusted fine and now they are best of friends.

You can transform your children's lives and world by the words of your mouth. Speak to create life, good health, long life, prosperity, abundance today and always. Thank you.

Disclaimer:

The information and opinions expressed here are believed to be accurate and based on the best judgement available to the author. Readers who fail to consult with appropriate health authorities assume the risk of any injuries. In addition, the information and opinions expressed here do not necessarily reflect the views of all health practitioners. The international health support group Acknowledges occasional differences in opinion and welcomes the exchange of different viewpoints. This entity is not responsible for users' errors, omissions or failures to consult their doctors for their necessary health needs. Thank you.